Endometriosis Diet

Signs, Symptoms and Treatment

Change Your Diet to Reduce impact

Theresa Bason

Table of Contents

Chapter 1: What is Endometriosis?

Endometriosis is a painful condition that can greatly impact your quality of life. Diet changes are said to help relieve symptoms, but does the evidence support these claims?

Endometriosis occurs when tissue that's normally found inside the uterus grows in other parts of the body. Tissue deposits (called implants) are most often found in the pelvis, but can also be found in more distant organs like the liver and the brain.

Endometrial tissues normally build up in the uterine lining each month until the lining is shed during the menstrual period. For various reasons, these cells are found in other parts of the body in women with endometriosis, causing chronic inflammation, scarring at affected sites, and heightened pain levels.

When I was first diagnosed with endometriosis, there was an air of casualness about the whole thing. I was told it probably wouldn't come back and, naturally, I thought the same.

While waiting for my second laparoscopy, I started to grasp the impact of endometriosis on my body and began experimenting with diet. Given that endometriosis is an inflammatory disease the endometriosis diet, therefore, requires eliminating or reducing foods that are known to increase inflammation, including:

Sugar
Gluten
Red meat
Dairy
Alcohol
Caffeine

In addition, research has shown that women with endometriosis often have higher levels of estrogen, and that estrogen can encourage tissue growth. This type of diet can help support the liver, which eliminates excess estrogen from the body, and it can also help stabilize hormones thanks to certain nutrients in the food.

Nutritionists such as Henrietta Norton suggest that the hormones used in meat production have an additional negative effect on our own hormones, by making their way into our body when consumed.

Norton's book, "Take Control of Your Endometriosis," includes compelling statistics from research showing that "women who ate green vegetables 13 times or more per week (roughly twice a day) were 70 per cent less likely to have endometriosis than those who ate green vegetables less than six times per week."

Though the diet may sound scary at first, it doesn't have to be about forceful restriction. In the beginning, you could just try cutting down a little on whatever you feel you might be eating slightly too much of, or whatever triggers your pain the most.

A common question I'm asked is, "So what do you eat?" But the truth is, I eat a lot. Cooking for the endometriosis diet doesn't have to be a problem once you've got to grips with what ingredients to buy.

In the U.S., and from my understanding, all over, vegan and gluten-free food options are growing. I know personally it's become much easier for me to shop at my local supermarket, but my favorite option (and one I really don't do enough) is online. With online shopping, you rarely have the issue of an item being out of stock or not being sold at a local supermarket, and you get a larger choice. Generally, my shopping list usually includes:

* Rice
* Quinoa

* Fruit and vegetables
* Rice pasta and noodles (or alternatives like lentil pasta, buckwheat
  noodles, etc.)
* Beans and pulses
* Gluten-free bread such as wraps, pita bread, and loaves
* Gluten-free oats
* Treats like raw dark chocolate and vegan ice cream, often made
  from coconut milk or cashew nuts
* Nuts, seeds, and dried fruit like coconut chips
* Herbs and spices
* Health foods such as cacao powder

Quite honestly, without the internet, I wouldn't have had any idea of where to start with gluten-free vegan cooking, but there are so many amazing blogs out there now that the problem has become a lack of time to try them all!

Some of the most influential bloggers I follow - who have made the endometriosis diet creative, enjoyable, and accessible - are Jessica Murnane, Ella Mills, Heather Crosby and Dana Shultz. These women have everything from quick, 30-minute meals to birthday cakes and decadent brunches.

Eating out can obviously pose its difficulties. I've flirted with the endometriosis diet for many years before fully committing, mainly because I told myself it was too hard to eat out with friends and not be fussy.

I'm not saying it's easy, but since committing to being gluten-free and dairy-free all the time, it's actually become much easier to make choices, and I've become much more confident in speaking to waiters about my requirements.

I still go to the places where I know I can eat everything and anything, and those are, of course, my favorite places to go. But now, if a friend wants to go for a pub lunch, I know how to handle it. My answer? Order the sides. I've had some pretty good meals made up of all of the bits I can eat and throwing them together.

Each one of us is affected differently by endometriosis and there is no one-size-fits-all when it comes to treatment, conventional or alternative. The endometriosis diet may not have the same effects on you as it has on me; it's not for everyone and that's OK. But leading a healthier lifestyle where possible is always a positive choice. So, even if it's just about getting a better night's sleep or topping up on your vegetable portions, the endometriosis lifestyle and diet could help support body and mind.

Chapter 2: Endometriosis Symptoms and Causes

Endometriosis Symptoms

Some women with endometriosis have no symptoms.

In fact, it's often discovered during medical tests or surgeries for other conditions.

However, most women experience symptoms that significantly affect quality of life, including:

* Pelvic or lower back pain
* Painful menstrual periods (dysmenorrhea)
* Heavy menstrual periods
* Pain during intercourse
* Painful bowel movements or urination
* Fatigue
* Bloating
* Digestive Distress (constipation, diarrhea, or nausea)

Endometriosis affects up to 10% of women and causes tissue that's normally found in the uterus to build up in other parts of the body. Symptoms include pain, heavy menstruation, digestive distress, fatigue, and bloating.

It's typically seen in women of childbearing age, but symptoms may persist into menopause or after hysterectomy if estrogen levels are high enough.

Up to half of affected women also struggle with infertility, but it's not known whether endometriosis causes infertility or is just associated with it.

Endometriosis Causes

Endometriosis is thought to be caused by a combination of genetic, physiologic, immune, and environmental factors. In fact, studies have found that a woman's risk increases by up to 7 times if her mother or sister has it. However, not everyone with a family history will develop the disease. Other factors appear to increase the likelihood of endometriosis.

One of the most common theories is retrograde menstruation, which occurs when endometrial cells and menstrual blood travel upward via the fallopian tubes. From there, the cells can implant into the abdominal lining and onto the organs, causing inflammation and scarring.

Nearly all women experience some degree of retrograde menstruation, but it's been suggested that a higher volume of blood enters the abdomen in women with endometriosis.

Is Endometriosis an Autoimmune Disease?

Recent research also suggests the immune system could greatly influence disease onset and severity. Autoimmune disease develops when the body's immune system mistakenly attacks healthy tissues.

Endometriosis shares several key features with autoimmune disease, including systemic inflammation and the presence of autoantibodies. There's also a strong overlap between endometriosis and other autoimmune conditions, like celiac disease and Graves' disease.

These similarities have many experts asking whether endometriosis should be classified as an autoimmune disease instead. It's an emerging area of research that will likely be explored in greater depth in coming years.

Chapter 3: Diet and Endometriosis

There's no known cure for endometriosis. The condition is commonly treated with surgery, hormone therapy, and medications.

No diet has been proven to treat endometriosis either. However, small studies and patient reports suggest that certain diet strategies can help reduce disease risk and lessen symptoms. This could be because certain foods can help control inflammation and influence levels of certain hormones.

These include omega-3 fats, vegetables, and other foods, which will be discussed below.

Replace Trans Fats with Omega-3 Fatty Acids

Significant research has looked at whether fat consumption affects endometriosis risk and symptoms. Unfortunately, some studies have found high-fat diets to be more beneficial, while others have found low-fat diets to be better. It's a tricky area for researchers because fat quality is likely just as important as quantity, perhaps even more so.

Omega-3 fatty acids appear to be especially beneficial, while trans fats are thought to increase risk. In one study of nearly 71,000 women:

* Women who ate the most trans fats were 48% more likely to have endometriosis than women who ate the least.

* Women who ate the most fats from animal products - and especially palmitic acid - had a 20% higher prevalence of endometriosis than those who ate the least.

* Women who ate the most omega-3 fatty acids were 22% less likely to have endometriosis than those who ate the least.

Even modest increases in omega-3 fat intake appear to be beneficial. One study found that replacing 1% of calories from trans fats with omega-3 fats decreases risk by 50%.

The exact mechanism for this is unknown, but omega-3 fats have been shown to reduce inflammatory chemicals in the body, including cytokines and certain types of prostaglandins.

For the record, trans fats are bad for you in many ways so replacing them with omega-3s makes sense regardless of whether you have endometriosis.

Aim to eat at least 7 ounces (about 200 grams) of fatty fish per week, and limit baked goods, fried foods, and packaged items.

Studies suggest that a diet higher in omega-3 fats and lower in trans fats may reduce endometriosis risk and severity. The recommendation for healthy adults of at least 7 ounces (about 200 grams) of fatty fish per week would also be beneficial for women with endometriosis.

Identify Food Intolerance and Eliminate Trigger Foods

Food intolerance foods can cause unpleasant reactions to specific foods. Common symptoms include digestive distress and skin rashes.

Small studies have found higher rates of food intolerance in women with endometriosis compared to healthy controls.

Troublesome foods vary widely from person to person, but these are the most common:

Gluten and Celiac Disease

Patient testimonials (reports) suggest that a gluten-free diet is effective in treating endometriosis.

This may be true, as some studies have shown an overlap between celiac disease and endometriosis.

This relationship isn't fully understood, but it's been proposed that chronic inflammation from celiac disease may trigger the onset of endometriosis.

A gluten-free diet may even provide symptom relief for those who don't have celiac disease.

In one study of 207 endometriosis patients, 75% of participants reported significant reductions in symptom severity after 12 months on a gluten-free diet. They also reported improved mental health, social function, vitality, physical function, and perceived healthiness after following the diet.

More studies are needed to understand the relationship between gluten and endometriosis. At the very least, those with celiac disease or a known sensitivity to gluten should strictly avoid it.

FODMAPs

FODMAPs are short-chain carbohydrates that are poorly digested in the small intestine.

They reach the colon largely intact and ferment in the gut, causing bloating, gas, abdominal pain, and other digestive symptoms for those who are intolerant of them.

Studies have established strong links between irritable bowel syndrome (IBS) and endometriosis.

A low FODMAP diet has been proven for treating IBS, and recent research suggests that it may be useful for easing endometriosis - related bowel symptoms as well. This is due in part to a high overlap rate between IBS and endometriosis.

In one study that included 58 women with both conditions, 72% of patients saw a great improvement in bowel symptoms after 4 weeks on a low FODMAP diet. The success rate for the low FODMAP diet was also significantly higher for women with endometriosis compared to women with just IBS.

Autoimmune Protocol

Research has shown strong links between endometriosis and autoimmune disease.

The Autoimmune Protocol (AIP) is a strict elimination diet designed for those with autoimmune disease. It's meant to correct imbalances in gut bacteria and reduce inflammation.

Unfortunately, there have been no scientific studies on it to date. But patients with various autoimmune diseases have reported symptom relief using the AIP in online forums.

Importantly, note that this diet is very restrictive. It's meant to be a short-term fix to help identify food intolerances for those with diagnosed autoimmune diseases.

If you have severe endometriosis and another autoimmune condition, a trial of the AIP may help after discussion with your doctor.

A gentler, easier alternative would be to keep a food and symptom journal for several weeks to identify foods that trigger symptoms.

There's a strong overlap between endometriosis and food intolerance. Gluten free or low FODMAP diets may be helpful in improving symptoms for some women. The autoimmune protocol may be helpful short-term for those who also have autoimmune disease.

Eat More Vegetables and Fiber

Everyone can benefit from eating more vegetables. Among many other advantages, higher vegetable consumption is linked to lower risk of endometriosis.

One large study of 504 women found risk to be significantly lower in women who eat a lot of green leafy vegetables. The mechanism for this isn't fully understood, but many vegetables are high in antioxidants, which help combat oxidative stress. Vegetables are also high in fiber which help body get rid of excessive estrogen.

In one study of 242 women, those who had the highest dietary fiber intake had significantly lower levels of estrone and estradiol (both forms of estrogen) than women who had the lowest fiber intake. The exceptions in this study were grapefruit and avocados, which were linked to higher estrogen levels.

Surprisingly, evidence is more mixed when it comes to endometriosis and fruit consumption. One study found higher fruit intake to increase risk, while other studies have found women who eat more fruit to have lower risk.

Aim for at least 5 servings of vegetables and 2 servings of fruit per day, endometriosis or not. Vegetables contain antioxidants, which may help reverse oxidative stress that comes with endometriosis.

Evidence is less clear on fruit intake, but most women would likely benefit from a couple of servings per day.

Endometriosis and Soy

Phytoestrogens and Soy are estrogen-like chemicals found in plants. Soybeans and soy products are the greatest dietary source, but phytoestrogens are also found in flax seeds, oats, fruits, herbs, and other foods.

A certain kind of phytoestrogen (called genistein) that's found in soy products has been said to help convert testosterone into estrogen. Since endometriosis is estrogen-dependent, some have questioned whether soy should be avoided.

Few studies have directly examined the relationship between soy and endometriosis, but limited data indicate it's neutral, and potentially even helpful.

In one study, women with higher concentrations of soy isoflavones in the urine were less likely to develop advanced endometriosis. This suggests that soy may help protect against the disease.

Evidence is not conclusive, but it seems that a high soy intake has no impact on the risk of developing endometriosis. Likewise, it probably does not make endometriosis any worse.

Don't Drink Too Much Alcohol

Moderate alcohol intake of up to 1 drink per day is generally considered safe for most women.

Beer, bourbon, and red wine contain phytoestrogens, which may convert to estrogen in the body. Just like soy, some have questioned whether they increase endometriosis risk.

Three large studies have found risk to be higher among women who drink the most alcohol, while 3 other studies found no link between alcohol and endometriosis

Notably, an often-cited study found that a compound found in red wine called resveratrol may limit the growth of endometrial tissue. But the study was conducted on mice, who were given very high doses of the compound. It wouldn't be possible to safely drink the amount of wine needed to see any benefit.

High alcohol intake causes many health problems, so it's best to limit yourself to 1 drink per day at most.

Several studies have found endometriosis risk to be higher among women who drink excessive alcohol, but other studies haven't shown a link. High alcohol intake, and especially binge drinking, has many negative health consequences. One drink or less per day is best.

Vitamins and Minerals for Endometriosis

Vitamins and Minerals have been reported to relieve symptoms common in endometriosis.

In many cases, studies on vitamins and minerals have used supplements rather than whole foods. As such, it's difficult to know the amounts of food that would yield similar benefits.

Antioxidant Vitamins

Antioxidants are compounds that protect against oxidative stress and cell damage.

Studies suggest that oxidative stress contributes to endometriosis onset and severity. Research also shows that the antioxidant vitamins C and E may provide symptom relief.

In one study of 59 women with pelvic pain and either endometriosis or infertility:

One group of 46 women received 1200 milligrams (mg) of vitamin E plus 1000 mg of vitamin C daily.
A second group of 13 women received placebo (fake) pills daily.

After 8 weeks, the vitamin group had significantly lower levels of known inflammatory markers compared to placebo.

Antioxidant Vitamins

Vitamin C is found in many fruits and vegetables and is particularly high in oranges. Vitamin E is found in foods like almonds and spinach.

Studies have also suggested that vitamin D may protect against endometriosis onset, although other studies have found it to have no significant effect on pain and other symptoms.

Vitamin D is found in fortified foods, fatty fish, and egg yolks.

More human studies are needed to know the safest and most effective vitamin doses for endometriosis. Speak with your doctor before beginning any new vitamin or supplement.

Iron

Women with endometriosis may be at higher risk for iron-deficiency anemia due to heavy menstrual periods. Symptoms include fatigue, dizziness, headache, shortness of breath, pale skin, weakness, irregular heart beat, and cold hands and feet.

A simple blood test can help determine if you're iron deficient. Your doctor may recommend supplements to help boost your iron levels. Diet changes can also help to improve iron status for those who are anemic. Red meat is rich in iron, although it's best not to consume fatty meats or large quantities of red meat.

Other diet sources of iron include seafood, nuts, green leafy vegetables, and fortified grain products.

For the record, the body absorbs iron from meat more effectively than from plant sources.

Thiamine

Vitamin B1 (thiamine) has been reported to ease menstrual pain.

One study of 556 young women with dysmenorrhea found that 100 mg of thiamine per day for 90 days completely relieved menstrual pain in 87% of volunteers and drastically reduced pain in 8% of volunteers.

Notably, this study didn't include women with endometriosis, and thiamine was in capsule form. But it's possible that it would help those with painful periods.

Know that thiamine deficiency isn't common among healthy women in industrialized nations. More research is needed to know if higher dose supplements would affect endometriosis.

The Recommended Dietary Allowance (RDA) is 1.1 mg per day for women (who aren't pregnant or lactating) and can be met by eating 3-5 servings of whole grains per day.

Magnesium

Magnesium is an element with many important functions in the body, including nerve and muscle regulation. It's available in many plant foods, including leafy greens, almonds, and beans. It's also available in capsule, powder, and lotion form.

Three small studies have found magnesium to be more effective in reducing menstrual pain than placebo. Few adverse effects were reported in these studies, but supplemental magnesium may cause diarrhea, drowsiness, or other symptoms in some.

Magnesium deficiency is quite common, with nearly half of Americans consuming less than the RDA. Magnesium supplements can help ensure that daily needs are met.

Summary:

Thiamine, magnesium, and vitamins C, D, and E have been reported to ease pain in endometriosis. Iron may be necessary for women with heavy periods. Ask your doctor if you might benefit from supplements.

Chapter 4: Complementary and Alternative Treatments for Endometriosis

Traditional Chinese Medicine

Traditional Chinese medicine (TCM) is used in many parts of the world as a complement to standard medical care.

It incorporates acupuncture, herbal treatments, massage, and other therapies. Patient testimonials indicate that TCM may provide symptom relief in endometriosis. But scientific evidence is somewhat limited.

Acupuncture

One review of 3 studies found that acupuncture improved pain and quality of life for volunteers. Women in this review received up to 16 treatments either once or twice a week for 15-25 minutes per session.

And another study of 67 women with endometriosis found acupuncture to greatly improve menstrual pain.

Acupuncture is generally well-tolerated with few side effects and may be worth a try for those dealing with pain.

Herbal Therapies

Herbal preparations have been used for centuries in Chinese medicine to treat various conditions.

One review of 2 small studies found traditional herbal preparations to reduce menstrual pain more effectively than hormonal drugs commonly used in endometriosis. No improvements were seen in rectal, back, or vaginal pain.

Herbal therapy isn't for everyone. Medicinal herbs interact with many medications and are not appropriate for those with certain health conditions.

The Punch Line

Endometriosis is largely influenced by hormonal and environmental factors that influence oxidative stress.

Since diet can protect cells against damage, alter hormone levels, and reduce inflammation, a change in eating habits may help lessen symptoms.

Several diet strategies are recommended:

* Eat fewer trans fats and more omega-3 fats. Limit baked goods, processed foods, and fried foods, and aim for 7 ounces (about 200 grams) of fatty fish per week.

* Avoid gluten if you have celiac disease or are sensitive to it.

* A trial of a low FODMAP diet is recommended if you suffer from bowel symptoms.

* Eat at least five servings of vegetables per day, including some leafy green veggies.

* Limit alcohol intake to 1 drink or less per day.

* Ask your doctor if you might benefit from supplemental thiamine, iron, magnesium, or vitamins C, D, E. Probiotics and melatonin

have also been reported to reduce endometriosis severity and are recommended with a doctor's approval only.

Endometriosis is a serious and painful condition, but lifestyle changes and the proper diet can greatly improve health and quality of life.

Chapter 5: Endometriosis Diet - Controlling the Symptoms Naturally

An endometriosis diet can be an integral part of managing the symptoms and pain caused by this disease. By making dietary changes, women with endometriosis are able to provide their bodies with the proper nutrients needed to control the causes of endometrial flare ups and the accompanying symptoms.

Endometriosis is a disease that has no diagnosed cause but the symptoms it causes are very real. The fact is that in women with endometriosis the symptoms and pain can be very debilitating. The endometrial tissue growing in the abdominal cavity can cause a number of health problems including inflammation, scarring, bleeding and infertility.

The aim of an endometriosis diet is twofold; one is to increase the overall health and immunity of the woman suffering from endometriosis and the second is to help limit the amount of estrogen and prostaglandins in her body.

Research has shown that women with healthy immune systems generally do not suffer from endometriosis. It is also known that endometrial cell growth is driven by estrogen and prostaglandins are thought to stimulate the body's production of estrogen.

Following a healthy endometriosis diet is a natural way to manage these issues and help with the painful symptoms that include cramps, inflammation, and bloating.

A woman's body is a complex living machine that is sensitive to the types of food she eats. In many cases certain food types can exacerbate an existing health problem while at the same time other food types can help mitigate or manage that same issue. With that in mind let's take a look at the two biggest culprits in the fight against endometriosis; estrogen and prostaglandins.

Avoiding foods that are high in saturated, mono-saturated and Trans fats is the first step to reducing the amount of estrogen stimulating "bad" prostaglandins present in the body.

Foods that are high in these types of dangerous fats include red meat, high fat dairy products and other products derived from animal fat such as lard. Instead opt for foods that are high in essential Omega-3 fatty acids such as fish oils, walnut oil, flax seeds oil and olive oil. These not only help reduce the "bad" prostaglandins but also have a relaxing effect on the uterine muscles.

It is also important to realize non-organic fatty foods and non-organic foods in general may also contain large amounts of PCB, dioxins and other Xenoestrogens that help contribute to the current estrogen dominance that many women are currently experiencing. When possible select foods that are organic in nature and wash all fruits and vegetables thoroughly before use.

Next on the list of good endometriosis diet ideas is incorporating more fiber into the woman's diet. Fiber is an integral part of any healthy diet and for women with endometriosis it is doubly so. Not only does help in the overall digestive process it is also instrumental in removing excess circulating estrogen. The recommended daily amount of fiber women should be ingesting is between 25 to 30 grams.

There are also foods that are believed to help regulate estrogen levels. They include mustard greens, broccoli, cabbage and turnips. It can be beneficial to eat one or two servings of these vegetables per day.

Cruciferous vegetables such as cabbage, sprouts, broccoli, cauliflower, kale and radishes are an important part of an endometriosis diet because they are high in B vitamins. B vitamins convert the form of estrogen known as estradiol to estriol. This is important because estriol is the form of estrogen that easily bonds to fiber and can be excreted from the body. These green leafy vegetables also contain magnesium which is known to help relax smooth muscle like found in the intestines and uterus.

There are also foods that should be avoided when planning an endometriosis diet; these include:

• Refined wheat products and sugars - wheat products contain phytic acid and gluten which can aggravate the symptoms of endometriosis. Refined sugars found in candy and chocolate can cause increased inflammation.

• Red meats, dairy products, and fried foods - these all contain large amounts of saturated fats that are known to increase the bad prostaglandins which stimulates estrogen production. There is also an increased risk to exposure to dioxins, pesticides, and other Xenoestrogens.

• Caffeine - in research studies caffeine increased estrogen levels and can increase abdominal cramping.

• Soy and soy protein products - foods made from soy contain large amounts of phytoestrogens which are believed to increase estrogen, the primary hormone responsible for its growth.

• Alcohol - while it's okay to have a drink every now and then excess alcohol consumption reduces vitamin B levels in the liver. Vitamin B is an essential vitamin in the removal of excess estrogen from a woman's body.

The dietary modifications needed for a successful endometriosis diet will take some work and planning. It is also important to understand

that it will take some time for your body to adjust and see the benefits
of using diet to help manage this disease.

Eating healthy means a healthy body, and a healthy body is able to
combat the effects endometriosis.

Chapter 6: Changing Lifestyle And Diet For Endometriosis

There is no denying that endometriosis can have a devastating effect on quality of life. Treatments for endometriosis vary between straightforward medication and surgery, but simple lifestyle changes should not be ruled out. A well compiled endometriosis diet, together with exercise can have a positive effect on the condition.

In the condition, the uterus lining tissue grows outside the uterus, with this external tissue reacting in exactly the same way as the uterus lining to the monthly variation of estrogen levels, provoking growth in response to high estrogen levels.

This is normal within the uterus, but when the tissue grows externally, serious pain can occur, with bleeding, leading to possible damage to organs, including the bowel and bladder. For some, the ultimate devastating effect can be infertility.

Medical science has progressed enough to know that conditions such as menstruation, menopause and fibroids, all estrogen reliant, are affected by lifestyle, diet and exercise. Most studies have concentrated on whether particular diets or activities are connected to endometriosis, with not much emphasis placed on whether those areas actually improved endometriosis symptoms.

However, it should not mean that they should be ignored. After all, since when did eating a proper balanced diet and taking sensible exercise do any harm.

Research has found that diets high in red meat and low in green vegetables and fresh fruit have a powerful link to endometriosis. This aligns well with other studies which have discovered similar links with this type of diet and fibroids and endometrial cancer.

So what conclusions can be drawn from this research?

One theory suggests that the fat within the diet manipulates production of prostaglandins by the body. These are chemicals that encourage contractions of the uterus and affect ovary function. It is widely believed that an increased level of prostglandins leads to more estrogen being produced, which in turn could influence endometrial tissue growth.

Other studies have concluded that the more fat consumed in the diet, then the higher the estrogen levels. This can occur in overweight people, and the likelihood is that overweight people will follow a high red meat, low fruit and vegetable diet. So the link is plain to see.

As far as exercise is concerned, it is already known that intense exercise causes women to have lighter periods, with greatly reduced production of estrogen. Studies carried out have found that regular, intensive physical activities leads to a big reduction in the chances of being diagnosed with endometriosis, with a definite improvement when exercise is performed more often.

What does this mean for the endometriosis sufferer?

Well, it is already evident that a proper diet and exercise can have a major effect on many conditions, so why not endometriosis? At the very least, you may well see a drastic difference in the severity of your endometriosis symptoms.

Whichever way you look at it, changing lifestyle and diet for endometriosis can only be a positive move.

Endometriosis Diet - Avoid These Foods And Improve Your Endometriosis Symptoms Naturally

If you are following an endometriosis diet, then you must know which foods to avoid to make a considerable difference to your symptoms. By simply being in control of what you eat, then the endometriosis symptoms can be improved.

The key to success is to form an endometriosis diet that eliminates foods that raise the level of prostaglandins. Prostaglandins are responsible for stimulating production of estrogen, the main culprit in inducing endometriosis symptoms such as menstrual cramps, heavy menstruation, nausea and vomiting amongst others.

The following are some of the foods that are best to avoid when following an endometriosis diet.

Sugar

All forms of sugar, whether artificial, refined or natural, can be responsible for the development of a more acidic situation within the body, which can provide encouragement for the inflammatory pain associated with endometriosis. Cutting down on sweeteners, sugary drinks and sweets, honey and chocolate is clearly advisable.

Caffeine

Consuming high amounts of caffeine-rich foods, such as coffee, tea and soda, is known to raise estrogen levels which can prompt endometriosis flare ups. Estrogen levels have been known to rise following consumption of more than two cups of coffee per day.

Wheat

Wheat contains both gluten and phytic acid, both of which can aggravate and increase painful endometriosis symptoms. Limited intake or total avoidance is the obvious option.

Dairy Products

Dairy foods, primarily milk and cheeses, encourage the production of prostaglandins, which cause a worsening of endometriosis symptoms. In order to maintain the required calcium levels, replacement sources need to be found, such as almonds, salmon and sardines.

Soy Products

Also contains phytic acid, but at higher levels than in wheat. Phytic acid aggravates the digestive system and causes a reduction in the absorption of minerals,such as calcium. Foods including soy are pasta, soy milk, granola- all best avoided.

Saturated Fats and Oils

Fatty acids stimulate the production of prostaglandins, and can be found in foods such as saturated fats, butter, margarine and fried foods. Best avoided or limited.

Refined Carbohydrates

Refined carbohydrates, found in white bread, flour, pastry, drain the nutritional reserves of the body. Better options are wholegrain breads, pasta and rice.

Alcohol

A properly functioning liver plays an important part in ridding the body of excess estrogen, helping with the control of endometriosis. Eliminating alcohol in the body can overwork the liver, reducing its ability to work efficiently.

Additives and Preservatives

Mostly found in processed and frozen food items. Ideally best to avoid when following an endometriosis diet as they can encourage increases in prostaglandins as well as general ill health.

Red Meat

Not only does meat induces prostaglandins production, but red meat may also contain growth hormones such as estrogen. Substitute protein-rich options such as walnuts, cashews, and sesame seeds should be considered in order to get the required protein intake.

The traditional endometriosis treatment offered by doctors, is to undergo hormone treatment or surgery. However, these options are not guaranteed to be successful, and can be expensive and perhaps more importantly, can lead to unwanted and potentially dangerous side effects. But, other options are available.

Many sufferers are choosing to take a more natural approach to their endometriosis treatment, finding it a far more palatable choice.

Chapter 7: What Is the Best Endometriosis Diet?

Women who are diagnosed with endometriosis must have some dietary modifications to help them cope. Certain foods can trigger the pain felt in endometriosis while some foods help you cope with pain and inflammation. We will start with an endometriosis diet recommendation that will help you control the symptoms of endometriosis.

Foods to take

Be sure to include these food types in your diet if you have endometriosis.

Fiber provides your body some elements that will help you cleanse your body with toxins, as well as help promote easy bowel elimination. It helps women who are suffering from endometriosis by reducing the level of estrogen that circulates in your body. It is important that these foods have to be certified organic. Eating organic food for endometriosis diet will ensure that you will take in fewer toxins that may worsen your condition. Examples of foods rich in fiber are:

- Fruits and vegetables

- Whole grains

- Brown rice

- Beans and legumes

Omega-3 fatty acids have a lot of good benefits to offer in endometriosis. It helps lessen the intensity of endometriosis symptoms aside from maintaining your nervous system and cardiovascular system. Foods rich in Omega-3 are the following:

- Tuna

- Any salt-water fish that has fat (salmon, sardines, herring)

- Sun flower oil

- Evening primrose

- Brazil nuts

- Olive oil

- Flaxseed

- Hemp seeds

- Pumpkin seeds

Foods to avoid

There are a lot of foods to avoid for endometriosis. Some of them may even contain your favorites. If you have endometriosis, you may notice worsening of signs and symptoms if you take these food types. If you are used to eating these foods, taper it off your diet or gradually reduce the amount you consume until you are used to not eating them. This will make sure that you have an endometriosis diet that does not promote worsening of symptoms. Foods to remove are:

- Wheat or foods rich in gluten such as breads, cakes and pasta.

- Processed foods must also be avoided as they contain many chemicals that can worsen your symptoms, not to mention gluten.

- Red meats, refined sugars, and honey promote production of prostaglandin that promotes pain and inflammation.

- Alcohol

- Coffee, tea, soft-drinks, or any beverage that contains caffeine.

- Chocolates

- Dairy products as it promotes inflammatory conditions
- Fried foods or any food that contains margarine and hydrogenated fats

- Soy products

Check what you eat and see if what you consume daily is a good for endometriosis diet that is programmed to help you live a comfortable life.

Is It Really Going to Help You Feel Better With Endometriosis?

When I first read the restrictions of the Endometriosis Diet, I really didn't think I could possibly stick to it. It seemed impossible and even unrealistic at the time. Thing is, my Endometriosis pain was not getting any better with my current diet and to be honest, I needed something to change.

I had another look at the diet and broke-down the basics of what it should include and exclude.

So, the inclusions should be:

* Heaps of good fats like Omega 3
* Heaps of berries, fruits and vegetables (especially greens)
* Use Exra Virgin Olive oil and Coconut Oil

Here's the tricky part......I was to exclude a whole bunch too!

Here are the exclusions:

* Dairy - Goats and Sheep products are okay
* Meat
* Sugar
* Gluten
* Preservatives, pesticides and fungicides
* No processed oils

So, to me this looked like there was not much left that I could actually eat! No cereal for breakfast! No toast for lunch! What do I put in my tea?

As I explored it all a little further, I discovered the reason WHY, I needed to cut them out. To me, I struggled to do anything unless someone gave me a real reason to do it. It was no good saying: cut this out and don't eat this because it is bad for your Endometriosis. This was just not enough motivation for me to cut all of these delicious things out of my life!

So, here is what I discovered:

1. Inflammation

Endometriosis is essentially an inflammatory condition. Our bodies are prone to inflammation. We are likely to have a swollen abdomen, bloating and suffer from other inflammatory conditions like bowel problems and interstitial cystitis. Dairy, Meat and Gluten are inflammatory in their nature. They encourage the hormone like substances called prostaglandins, which stimulate inflammation, clotting and pain. (Don't worry there are two other prostaglandins which do the opposite!)

This is also the reason we want to include heaps of Omega 3 into our diet. Omega 3 encourages the Prostaglandin 1 & 3, which reduce inflammation and pain. - definitely want to encourage those ones!

2. Immune system

Our immune system is low. This is a well known fact about Endometriosis. We want to build the immune system with good foods, highly nutritious foods and as much raw food as we can to get live enzymes into the body. Sugar reduces our immune system within minutes and one teaspoon of it will reduce it for hours. So, using a better alternative to sugar, like Stevia is much better for us.

3. Gluten intolerance and Endometriosis

Gluten intolerance is directly linked to much of the pain we have with Endometriosis. Gluten intolerance causes all sorts of problems. It can be the reason you suffer from low iron levels and various other mineral deficiencies. Gluten will also cause headaches, bloating and poor digestion.

4. Endometriosis and Dioxin, Xenoestrogens

Endometriosis is directly linked to dioxin, which is a toxin found in our environment. It may even be within some of our foods. Toxins of any description are bad for Endometriosis, which includes hair dyes and soaps. They play havoc with our endocrine system. - the hormone stuff. So, if you have endo, chances are you also have Oestrogen Dominance. All these substances in our environment and in processed foods contain them. Research some of the ingredients you eat each day and you will be amazed!

5. Processed oils

Basically, the process of extracting many of the oils we eat, is through heat. This process changes the molecular structure of the oil. This new shape, doesn't fit into our cells. They land up affecting our cell structure and giving our liver more toxins to process.

Use only Extra Virgin Olive Oil and Coconut Oil for cooking.

So, the Endometriosis Diet has its merits and there is now enough reason to stick to it. For me, it has been over a year of sticking to it!

I have had the odd bit of meat here and there but no dairy, sugar or gluten. The results have been amazing. I felt the change within a few months! I no longer have pain in my abdomen on a permanent basis!

Don't believe for a minute that what you eat doesn't make a difference.....because it does!

Chapter 8: Starting An Effective Endometriosis Diet That Eliminates The Potential For Candida Overgrowth

An effective endometriosis diet can have a significant impact on the pain and other common symptoms of endometriosis and may even help to regular and prevent Candida overgrowth. Numerous studies have shown that women who implement anti-Candida diets have received notable improvements in their issues with endometriosis.

This and other research has shown that strategic changes in eating habits can create increased levels of energy, regulate hormones and moods and reduce the discomfort of endometriosis and other reproductive or systemic ailments when implemented on a regular basis.

The Suspected Connection Between Candida And Endometriosis

Many medical experts have long suspected that there might be a connection between endometriosis and Candida. This is due in large part to the high prevalence of patients suffering from both Candida overgrowth and Endometriosis, though the determination of which infection is responsible for the development of the other has not been definitively established.

The presence of excessive amounts of Candida within reproductive areas can create the idea condition for hormonal imbalance, inflammation and other reproductive issues. The hormonal imbalances that are typical of patients who suffer from endometriosis can also be catalysts for a yeast infection. Thus, treating one with dietary changes such as the implementation of an endometriosis diet, will impact both conditions.

Foods To Avoid

In both instances women should begin to eliminate all red meat and dairy products from their diets. These tend to create excessive amounts of acid in the digestive process which can affect the digestive and reproductive systems causing constipation, indigestion and imbalances within the vagina, specifically those that create higher levels of susceptibility for a yeast infection.

Fatty, fried selections should be taken off of the list of foods to eat as well as canned foods, frozen foods and pre-packed or ready-made selections. These can overwhelm the body with toxins and prevent it from obtaining optimal levels of health. There are also fewer vital nutrients in these selections which make them virtually empty or unnecessary calories to consume. When making an effort to fight Candida as well as endometriosis, selections that are commonly thought to be healthy such as wheat and soy should be discontinued as well. These things can be eaten from time to time but must no longer be part of the routine diet.

Foods To Include

The basis of an endometriosis diet should be both simple and natural. The body will gain its best advantages through the consumption of organic selections such locally grown produce, whole grains and lean meats and fish. Selections such as broccoli and leafy green vegetables such as collard and turnip greens are known to naturally regulate female hormones and can provide a significant amount of punch in the fight against endometriosis.

What You Need to Know About the Endometriosis Diet

It is a must that we understand this condition known as Endometriosis before you delve into the right diet to go with it. Endometriosis is a condition that is estrogen - sensitive and is characterized by the painful menstrual cramping that happens and is largely due to the prostaglandin synthesis in the body.

To further explain, prostaglandins are naturally occurring fatty acids and are derived by the body from food intake and the body has the ability to produce different types of prostaglandins through a maze of different body processes.

Now, the right endometriosis diet helps block the bad prostaglandins and their negative actions to the body and increases the good prostaglandins to do the exact good opposite to the body. Bad prostaglandins causes uterine contractions which results to great pain during the menstrual cycle.

It is also important to minimize or totally eliminate the intake of the leading causes of the production of more bad prostaglandins such as saturated fats, butter, animal meat, and lard.

Apart from totally getting rid of the bad prostaglandin boosters, you must also increase the intake of fibrous foods like oats, wheat, and other grains.

Fiber is not only helpful for digestion; it also decreases the total estrogens that circulate the body. There is a much fiber found in beans, brown rice, vegetable and also fruits. To control and modulate the body's estrogen levels, you need to eat broccoli, cabbage, and turnips.

At the same time, you also need to get away from red meat that promotes negative prostaglandins, carbohydrates found in flour and cakes, refined sugar, alcohol that uses the stock vitamin B in the liver, caffeine which is found in tea and coffee, soda that increases abdominal cramps, chocolate due to its high level of sugar, milk and cheese, fried foods, soy products, canned goods and anything that has additives or preservatives.

Nothing beats the intake of vitamins and minerals through a well balanced diet and the endometriosis diet requires the intake of as many vitamins and minerals as possible. However, if we do not watch the food that we eat, we may end up eating a lot of food that would aggravate the endometriosis condition even more.

Endometriosis diet will result in lot of changes in the eating habits so you have to be ready to undergo this challenging diet or else you won't be able to stop this painful condition and may even worsen it.

Chapter 9: How To Be Successful On The Endometriosis Diet

Remember that well-known saying, "you are what you eat?" Well, for most endometriosis sufferers, the familiar phrase holds all the wisdom in the world.

Hurting month after month from endo, the uncomfortable signs and symptoms associated with your menstrual cycle oftentimes read like your favorite horror story:

• severe belly cramping
• fatigue
• heavy menstruation flow
• backaches
• mind-numbing headaches

Leaving you exhausted, frustrated and miserable, especially when there is no known "cure" for this crippling situation that impacts over 5.5 million women in North America alone.

What Is Happening To My Body?

When you have your period and the cellular material that lines the uterus gets ready to exit, problematic tissues (a.k.a. endometrial tissue) sometimes find their way outside of the uterus yet act the same way, expanding and spasming in preparation for menses. The issue is that they are now kept in and around the pelvic area (i.e. your fallopian tubes, ovaries, bladder, etc.) with nowhere to go. The soreness triggers the painful periods you experience.

Endometriosis is a hormonal ailment that is directly impacted by estrogen levels. In fact, many other feminine reproductive issues like fibroids, ovarian cysts, PCOS, inability to conceive and the like are all found to be the result of an estrogen imbalance in the body.

You Are What You Eat

The great news is you can gain control over and handle endometriosis by simply eating better. Sounds too good to be true? We can call this the Endometriosis Diet, but "Fibroid Buster," "Ovarian Cyst Diet," "Diabetes Miracle" or any other degenerative disease can be substituted because when it's all said and done, the body is merely doing the best it can with the fuel we give it. Garbage In = Garbage Out.

Fortunately for us though, your system is forgiving enough to give us warning signs before it completely breaks down and you are here because you've heard the warning signs and want to take action to reverse the damage and prevent further damage.

By reduction of certain foods that promote prostaglandin you can effectively reduce and eliminate painful signs and symptoms like excessive menstrual cramps, heavy hemorrhaging, nausea, queasiness and diarrhea in as little as one to two cycles and never have another occasion or outing ruined by a crippling visit from your monthly menses.

Regrettably, the typical American diet relies far too heavily on comfort foods. Chips, sodas, french fries and animal meat make up the greater part of our daily intake of food, with not a colorful vegetable in sight unless you consider the ketchup put on your burger a part of the vegetable family. So it does take commitment to make the dietary changes your body is frantically calling out for.

To make it simpler to get around the grocery store aisles on your future visit, here are the top 10 foods to avoid while following an Endometriosis Diet:

Dairy Products
Refined Sugar
Meat
Alcoholic beverages
Wheat
White Flour Products (i.e. cakes, cookies, pasta, white rice, etc.)
Soy Byproducts
Caffeine
Saturated Fats & Oils
Refined Foods

So you're probably thinking, 'well, what CAN I eat then?' That is a sensible question so I will give you a straightforward answer. A good rule of thumb when you are out store shopping is to just stay along the perimeter of the supermarket. Generally speaking, this is where the fresh fruits and vegetables are featured. If you follow this rule of thumb you are also less likely to be persuaded by the frozen ice cream sandwiches and cakes attractively displayed in the center aisle sand won't even realize that they are on sale two for five dollars this week!

Nutritious Substitutes You May Not Have Looked Into:

Sugar - Agave Nectar
Soy Sauce - Bragg'-s Liquid Aminos
Dairy Milk - Almond Milk
Butter - Flaxseed Oil (can be used to "butter" your bread, flaxseed shouldn't be heated)
Table Salt - Sea Salt
Seasoned Salt - Fresh Herbs (cilantro tastes great with just about everything)
Bottled Juice - Freshly Juiced Fruits & Vegetables
Peanut Butter - Almond Butter
Potato Chips -Flaxseed Chips
Dairy Cheese - Rice Cheese
Meats - Beans

Milk Chocolate - Dark Chocolate

Although it will probably be challenging at first, eventually you will get used to eating with a fresh new perspective and even notice your taste buds changing as you start craving more endo-friendly foods. It is more of a life-style change than a diet but it is absolutely achievable. Just like any new habit, you will get better with time and practice.

It's All in the Food - Endometriosis and Vegan Diet

There is a great connection between endometriosis and the vegan diet. The treatment of endometriosis must take into account the relief of symptoms as well as the underlying causes. In this case, the balance of the hormones progesterone and estrogen must be done.

The treatment should aim to reduce or increase these hormones in the body and to do so, dietary changes must be considered. If you make certain dietary changes, it can improve your endometriosis significantly.

Both the vegan diet and the endometriosis diet recommend eliminating red meat and dairy which are great contributors of inflammation in your body.

A vegan diet is a type of vegetarian diet that excludes dairy products, eggs, meat and any other animal derived ingredients. This also includes foods processed using animal products as well.

Most vegans will also avoid products that have been tested on animals or non-food products that are derived from animals including wool, fur and leather, however this is not a requirement with the endometriosis diet.

The vegan diet includes all beans, legumes, fruits, grains and vegetables as well as all the foods you can create by combining them. There are also vegan versions of foods such as ice cream, vegan mayonnaise, cheese and hot dogs.

There are many similarities between both diets. The good news is that you can use recipes from the vegan diet as well as recipes from the endometriosis diet as they follow very similar principals.

The foods encouraged for both diets include fresh and organic fruits and vegetables. These will benefit you in various ways. Foods such as artichokes, kale, cauliflower, beets and broccoli work by supporting the work of the liver.

The liver's work is to break down estrogen in the body. If it does not work properly, then it is unable to eliminate estrogen causing a build up of it, which makes endometriosis worse. Additionally fiber which will come from the fruits and vegetables consumed, allows your body to excrete excess estrogen through the digestive system and reduce the recirculation of hormones in the body. Not only that, if you suffer from constipation, then fiber will help process your food a lot faster.

Following a diet plan like this produces less estrogen circulating within the body which reduces the symptoms of endometriosis as well as the chances of developing it for those who are not current sufferers.

Although a vegetarian diet will reduce endometriosis signs and symptoms, an important meat that can help is cold water fish caught in the wild such as salmon. This is because it contains essential omega 3 fatty acids that when added to the your diet can reduce inflammation.

When deciding to go on an endometriosis and vegan diet it is important to consider that dairy is not necessarily helpful to your condition. A good example is with yogurt, where cows are given hormones to keep them lactating even when they are not pregnant.

These hormones are passed on to you when you eat dairy products like yogurt, milk or cheese, creating an imbalance in your own hormones. Additionally, yogurt that is commercially made has gelatin that comes from the by-products of animals such as the hooves.

It is therefore better that your diet has foods like kale which has 70% of the amount of calcium found in milk, rather than dairy products. Other sources of non animal calcium include raw sesame and even molasses.

Another advantage of the endometriosis and vegan diet is that you avoid the antibiotics used in commercial livestock production. These are found in the production of poultry, pork, lamb and beef.

The antibiotics are given to the animals to protect against disease or as immunization. However, they are not all passed out of the body but remain in the meat and especially fat of the animal. This means that you consume these when you eat meat. According to studies done, these products lower our immunity against cancer and other diseases as well.

Overall there is a lot you can do to get rid of your endometriosis symptoms and diet can account for up to 70% of the changes in your body. A diet that follows the principles of the endometriosis diet and vegan diet is one of the best ways to go to improve your health all round.

Chapter 10: You Are What You Eat

As we already know, Endometriosis is a serious condition that affects women. It occurs when tissues similar to the endometrial stroma and glands that line the uterus, show up in other areas of the body, instead of only existing within the uterus.

These rebel tissues are known as endometriosis lesions, and are usually found anywhere within the pelvic region (IE. Fallopian tubs, ovaries, pelvic sidewall, etc.). Due to the prime location of the endometriosis lesions, the most common symptom of this medical condition is pelvic pain.

While many women seek medical therapy, others find that by simply controlling their diet they are successfully living a symptom free life.

How can a diet improve endometriosis symptoms?

An endometriosis diet works to relieve and/or prevent some of the severe symptoms experienced during menstruation such as:

* Backache

* Fatigue

* Severe cramping

* Menorrhagia (heavy menstrual bleeding)

* Dysmenorrhea (pain or discomfort)

* Dyspareunia (pain in the pelvic or vaginal region during intercourse)

The objective of a controlled diet is to reduce estrogen levels, increase the body's energy level, relieve painful cramps, normalize hormones and stabilize emotions.

It has become evident that endometriosis is an estrogen-sensitive condition. However, the severe cramping that a woman experiences, is typically a result of prostaglandin synthesis in her body.

Prostaglandins are fatty acids that naturally occur from dietary phospholipids. Prostaglandins can be broken down into three separate groups:

1. Prostaglandin E1 (PGE1) - This form helps to relieve symptoms of endometriosis

2. Prostaglandin E2 (PGE2) - This form encourages menorrhagia

3. Prostaglandin F2a (PGF2a) - This form can lead to nausea, vomiting and diarrhea.

Essentially, when combined, PGE2 and PGF2a create the severe symptoms women who suffer from endometriosis experience during menstruation. However, the right change in diet can actually block the production of PGE2 and PGF2a and increase the production of PGE1 to help overcome symptoms.

The following is how such a diet can be achieved.

Fatty acids: It is known that fatty acids such as saturated fats, lard, butter and animal and organ meet increase the amount of PGF2a that is produced, while omega-3 fatty acids such as evening primrose oil, flax seeds and oil, pumpkin seeds, sunflower oil and walnut oil increase production of PGE1. Therefore, when a woman decreases the amount of "bad fat" in her diet, she will experience positive results.

Fiber: Aside from decreasing the intake of bad fat, women seeking dietary treatment for their endometriosis should have a diet high in fiber. A high fiber diet (approximately 25 grams per day) can reduce the amount of circulating estrogens. Good sources of fiber are beans, brown rice, fruits and vegetables, oatmeal and whole grains.

Dairy: Just like bad fats can increase symptoms, so can diary products. Unfortunately, dairy is a fantastic source of calcium. Therefore, if a woman chooses to eliminate diary from her diet, she needs to find other calcium sources by either taking supplements or eating foods that contain the mineral such as almonds, dark green veggies (IE. spinach, kale, broccoli, etc.), Figs, sesame seeds, etc. Other food that should be avoided during menstruation includes caffeine, chocolate, alcohol, fried foods, salt, sugar and refined carbohydrates (IE bread, cake, pastries, pasta, etc.)

Depending on what a woman feels needs to be eliminated from her diet during menstruation, she may need to consider taking supplements in order to maintain a healthy diet. Before taking supplements, women should consult their doctor.

Chapter 11: Achieving Pregnancy Through Natural Endometriosis Treatment

It is estimated that 10%-15% of women suffer from some level of endometriosis at some point in their lives, but many women are unaware of what exactly endometriosis is and how it can lead to infertility.

Endometriosis involves the implantation of endometrial tissue outside of the uterine walls. Its causes are not entirely understood, but this tissue can implant itself throughout the reproductive system, as well as throughout the body. It wreaks havoc on the implantation locations, leading to scar tissue and adhesions that can cause pain and other serious complications for the rest of a woman's life.

Endometriosis is one of the leading causes of infertility, and women who suffer from it are also exposed to varying degrees of pain (both during the cycle and day to day) and other unbearable symptoms.

Women often experience extreme bloating, and pain during intercourse as well as urination and bowl movements. Typical endometriosis treatment involves invasive surgical procedures and hormone alteration. The hormones that the medical community often prescribes typically come with their own set of side effects, and are often very hard on a women's body.

The worst part is that even when a woman subjects herself to all of that, she will still be told that there is no endometriosis cure and that she will likely have to deal with the repercussions of her endometriosis throughout her life.

Endometriosis infertility is one of the most difficult symptoms for many women dealing with endometriosis, and for a woman trying to get pregnant, endometriosis can often be one of the most painful obstacles she has to overcome.

Endometriosis is known to damage the fallopian tubes and ovaries, and even in mild cases it often makes conceiving more difficult than it should be. Achieving an endometriosis pregnancy can often seem like an impossible task, but there is endometriosis help for women willing to pursue an endometriosis natural treatment.

While the medical community is unaware of any endometriosis cure, the endometriosis treatments available there are often more difficult to handle than the endometriosis itself.

However, by following a set diet, endometriosis sufferers often find that they are able to control their endometriosis symptoms effectively on their own, and even go on to achieve an endometriosis pregnancy.

The endometriosis diet is aimed at reducing estrogen levels in the body naturally without hormonal injections or intervention. Many women have found great success by incorporating these changes into their day to day routine, and if you are suffering from endometriosis infertility this may be the most non-invasive way for you to achieve that endometriosis pregnancy you have long dreamed of.

Endometriosis and Pregnancy - Beating the Odds

Endometriosis and pregnancy are two inter-related health conditions that millions of women of child bearing age struggle with every year. The simple fact is endometriosis can and will make conceiving a child more difficult in most instances. This does not mean a woman cannot get pregnant but it can throw a monkey wrench in the process.

Exactly how endometriosis affects a woman's chance at pregnancy is not fully known but studies that have been conducted into the issue show that she is less likely to conceive then a woman who does not suffer from this disease. These studies have shown that about twenty percent of women with endometriosis will be unable to conceive and that of all infertile women twenty one to forty four percent have this disease.

What isn't known is why endometriosis affects a woman's ability to conceive a child. Is it the endometriosis itself or is there something else at work in conjunction with it.

The path to getting pregnant for women with endometriosis varies. Many women get pregnant naturally without any outside medical help. For women who are struggling with endometriosis and pregnancy it is important that they talk with their doctor /gynecologist about medical interventions that may help increase their chances of conceiving a child.

Women with endometriosis who are trying to get pregnant naturally may increase their odds if they consider the following:

1. Get started early in life - Studies have shown that women in their twenties are more likely to get pregnant then women in their thirties and older. Since endometriosis is shown to interfere with a woman's fertility, it will continue to make conceiving harder the older she gets.

2. Get healthy - Many women have success in managing their condition when eating an endometriosis diet. A healthy diet, combined with regular exercise, can help minimize the effects of endometrial growths and provides her body with the necessary nutrients to successfully nourish an embryo.

If after a period of six months to a year a woman has still not gotten pregnant naturally she can turn to her gynecologist or infertility specialist for help. There are several treatment or procedure options available to help increase the chance for a successful pregnancy.

1. Laparoscopic endometriosis surgery - This minimally invasive surgical procedure is done to diagnose endometriosis and also to cut and remove endometrial growths from the abdominal organs. This type of surgery is not a cure but it can provide a window in which a woman can successfully conceive. Studies do indicate that laparoscopic surgery can increase the likelihood of a successful pregnancy.

2. Fertility drugs - The use of drugs such as Clomid and Serophene can help stimulate ovulation in women who are having difficulty conceiving.

3. In Vitro Fertilization (IVF) - IVF is an assisted reproductive technique that has shown good results in women with endometriosis and pregnancy issues. It should be noted that the success rate of IVF for women with endometriosis is about half that of other women with infertility issues.

There are risk factors for pregnant women with endometriosis that can lead to serious complications during their pregnancy. A recent study by medical researchers in Sweden found that women with endometriosis are at a higher risk for the following:

1. Premature Birth -Women with endometriosis are at higher risk for having their baby's preterm. They also found that women who also underwent IVF procedures to become pregnant were at an even greater risk for preterm birth then women who did not.

2. Pre eclampsia - This is high blood pressure that develops in pregnant women during their second and third trimester. Women with endometriosis are at a higher risk for developing this dangerous condition that also includes protein in their urine and an increased risk for post birth.

3. Caesarean Section - In the study it was found that almost twice as many women with endometriosis had their babies delivered via C-section. It was also discovered that these women had a higher incidence of induced premature birth then spontaneous premature birth. The researchers conducting the study have theorized that complications with the placenta may be at the root of it.

It is estimated that over 9 million women worldwide suffer from endometriosis. Every year a good percentage of these women get pregnant and deliver healthy babies. With the proper medical support and care it is possible to beat the odds that this disease presents. Just remember that endometriosis and pregnancy are not mutually exclusive.

Chapter 12: Do You Have Endometriosis and Inflammatory Bowel Syndrome?

Many women who have Endometriosis also have another ailment called Inflammatory Bowel Syndrome (IBS). And on the flip side, many women present with an inflamed bowel will find out that it has been caused by Endometriosis.

This is where the endometrial tissue grows out of the uterus and onto the bowel causing many bowel symptoms. It has been found that as many as 60% of women with an Endometriosis diagnosis also suffer from IBS.

Endometriosis and IBS is so common that in a study done, 25% of the patients surveyed suffered from painful bowel movements and intestinal cramping. 35% suffered from constipation and a further 60% suffered from frequent diarrhea.

Both illnesses cause symptoms that include constipation, intestinal cramping, abdominal pain, painful bowel movements, diarrhea, alternating between diarrhea and constipation, vomiting and nausea, rectal bleeding and rectal pain as well.

Some people suffering from these conditions may only have one symptom, but others tend to have more than one. The condition tends to become worse during your period or prior to having your period. It can be quite frustrating because sometimes, even after running several tests nothing is found.

For most patients, Endometriosis is not found on the bowel directly. However, 10-15% of women suffering from this condition have it on their bowel directly. If Endometriosis is found on the bowel, surgery can be the solution. Often a laparoscopy will be done to take care of the Endometriosis and inflammatory bowel syndrome where the outer layer of the bowel is peeled off.

In some cases the layer that is below the top layer may have to be cut to ensure that the condition is treated effectively. It is then sewn over to maintain the integrity of your bowel wall reducing the symptoms of both Endometriosis and IBS.

In severe cases more significant surgery may be required. If so, then a bowel resection may be the solution to treat the problem completely.

How Is It Diagnosed?

If you suspect that you have Endometriosis and Inflammatory Bowel Syndrome, seek advise from your Doctor immediately. He or She can do a range of tests to diagnose both Endometriosis and separately IBS. There is a lot that you can do to manage both of these illnesses and an earlier diagnosis can help you immensely with the time it takes to start healing. A good place to start would be to look at your diet. The Endometriosis Diet is a great place to look at as the diet is designed to also minimize the most common symptoms of Inflammatory Bowel Syndrome.

Diet and Endometriosis: Why Red Meat Is a No-No

When it comes to endometriosis, diet is all-important, and red meat is a no-no. But why? Well, before that question is answered, it is perhaps better to look at the condition itself and find out what causes it.

Endometriosis is a condition that affects only women and is manifested in the uterus region of the body. The uterus itself is lined with endometrial cells that are known as womb cells. What happens in a normal woman is that these cells build up, and then during menstruation, they void themselves, leaving the uterus clean, and thus the cycle begins again.

Endometriosis, however, is when the lining of the uterus does not void itself, and settles in areas outside the uterus such as the lower pelvis. It can cause lesions on the muscle.

For the women who experience this, it can be very painful. The symptoms are characterized by constant pelvic pain, a gnawing pain in the thighs, trouble walking, trouble going to the bathroom and very painful sex and infertility.

There is no cure as such for the disease. However, there are ways in which the symptoms can be improved. You can undergo surgery every so often in order to remove the excess cells. Along with this, you can also go on hormonal therapies or use lots of pain medication.

The homeopathic way

Aside from resorting to normal medicine, you can also try to manage the symptoms on a homeopathic level. One of the ways in which to do this is to control the diet that you eat. One often underestimates just how much you can actually do if you simply try and eat the correct diet for the ailment that you are struggling with.

In the case of endometriosis, one of the main things to steer clear of is, without a doubt, red meat. The reason for this is that medical research has shown that the consumption of red meat leads to more prostaglandins building up in your system.

These are many complex fatty acids that are generally present in your body, but eating red meat generates more of them. They are also responsible for period cramps and other such things.

The prostaglandins bond with oestrogen in your body, causing the endometrial cells to grow, as they are fed by the process of oestrogen synthesis. This is the reason why in order to alleviate your endometriosis, you should stop eating red meat right away.

If you can control one thing, make sure that it is your diet, because you do not want to find yourself in a position where you suffer from this type of condition for longer than necessary.

Chapter 13: The Benefits of a Good Diet Plan for Endometriosis

Endometriosis is a disorder of the female reproductive system. Although this has nothing to do with the organs itself, the menstrual cycle as well as the female hormones associated with menses triggers the development and ongoing formation of endometriosis. The pain comes from the inflammation and adhesions that form as a result of endometrial tissue growing outside of the uterus. So, can a good diet plan for endometriosis ease the problems?

There are a number of theories behind the cause of endometriosis, including a mal-functioning immune system. The immune system is in place to eliminate any foreign elements within our bodies. For women with endometriosis the immune system either can't tackle the endometrial tissue that occurs outside of the uterus or it doesn't recognized that it shouldn't be there.

To improve the immune system one of the most helpful exercises is a thorough evaluation of nutritional intake. By doing this and introducing a healthy diet women suffering from endometriosis can greatly reduce the severity of symptoms and ease pain.

Health practitioners say that even if there are many treatments available for endometriosis, nutrition and a good diet plan still play a major role.

The idea is that eating well does not just ease the pain and other symptoms, but can also help you achieve hormonal balance. Plus, a good diet plan designed to tackle endometriosis can also help lessen your estrogen level and prostaglandins.

With regards to symptoms, prostaglandin normally fueled by estrogen, is the main culprit in severe abdominal cramps and pain. These hormones are also in charge of the other symptoms such as diarrhea, menorrhagia, vomiting and nausea.

So the best way to start your endometriosis treatment alongside with the other means of medications is to come up with a good diet plan.

Keep reading for three diet tips to get you started on an endometriosis diet. For more information on what to eat and what to avoid sign up for the free newsletter below.

1. Cut back on caffeine:

Caffeine is a big-league trigger of symptoms, especially abdominal cramping and diarrhea. Caffeine is highly stimulating to the digestion of normal individuals, and if you have endometriosis, it can be a disaster. So it is best for people with endometriosis to do away with caffeinated products from their diet.

The most common sources of caffeine are coffee, tea and regular cola. To quit or reduce caffeine, health experts recommend that you reduce your intake of coffee, tea, and caffeine-containing colas by five ounces every five to seven days, until you are drinking no more than 100 to 120 milligrams of caffeine a day.

2. Eat foods rich in fiber:

Since painful bowel movements can be a symptom of endometriosis, it is a good choice to eat more foods rich in fiber.

Fiber is the wall, or cellulose portion, of every plant cell including grains, beans, fruits and vegetables. It is not digestible. Instead, it travels through the digestive tract into the large intestine or colon. Once the fiber reaches the intestine, it combines with water in your digestive tract to create softer stools. Hence, it will be easier for you to eliminate symptoms like constipation.

There is also a theory that a fiber rich diet can reduce the amount of estrogen in the body. The thought is that the fiber binds with the estrogen and carries it out of the body in the stools, however more research is needed to determine if this is the case.

Endometriosis and Diet - Garlic

Endometriosis growing somewhere else other than the endometrium also reacts to hormonal signals of the monthly menstrual cycle by building up tissue, breaking it, and eliminating it through the menstrual period. As we know garlic contains variety of nutrients that are important to women with endometriosis.

We will discuss how garlic effects women with endometriosis.

1. Immune system

Garlic is natural antioxidant that helps the immune system fighting against the forming of free radical and foreign invasion including bacteria, virus as well as forming of endometrial implants and adhesion.

2. Circulation system

Garlic is a blood thinner, it helps to strengthen the arterial wall and increase the blood circulation in the body including the abdomen resulting in lessening the heavy blood flow and menstrual pain during menstruation caused by over active uterine muscles.

3. Vitamin A

Vitamin A helps boost the immune system. It also helps to reduce heavy blood flow during menstruation.

4. Vitamin C

Vitamin C helps strengthen the capillary wall. It helps to increase the digestive function that is essential for women with endometriosis.

5. Calcium

Deficiency of calcium not only contributes to bone loss but also increases the risk of over active uterine muscles that cause menstrual pain.

6. Hormone balancing

Garlic containing substances help in stimulating the production of sex hormones which reduce the excessive amount of bad estrogen but also increases sexual desire for women with endometriosis.

Chapter 14: Do You Need An Ultrasound For Endometriosis?

Endometriosis can be a tricky to diagnose because it doesn't often show up when ultrasound and x-rays are done. There are some doctors who are really good at using ultrasound for detecting endometriosis, though even they will miss it at times. It often depends on the severity of the cases, where it is located, and if other conditions can be eliminated from consideration. While ultrasound for endometriosis can be a useful tool, it might often miss what is really going on.

The most common type of ultrasound used for detecting endometriosis is vaginal, but a rectal ultrasound may be used as well. This means a wand is inserted into the vagina (or rectum). A scanner is then moved across the belly. The sound waves that are used will form a picture or video of the area. The pictures can then be studied for some of the signs of this condition.

Ultrasound normally comes after the physical examination and if there are unanswered questions about what the problem you are having. Though there are times when the ultrasound will easily detect the presence of endometriosis, there is also the possibility that the ultrasound will fail.

Either way, after this procedure is completed, a patient might then be scheduled for laparoscopy. This involves a small, lighted camera that is inserted in through the belly button or through small incisions near the pubic area. This can be used for a closer view of your reproductive or internal organs. The places affected can then be treated after a biopsy of any suspicious tissues is done.

Some doctors might view ultrasound for endometriosis as a standard part of the search for the condition, while others may think it is not effective enough to be relied upon. Most will still do it, as there is always hope they may notice something this way.

Either way, a person should remember that just because there was nothing found via the ultrasound, that does not mean that they do not have endometriosis. Further evaluation should always be done to be sure.

Chapter 15: How Can I Avoid a Hysterectomy for Endometriosis and What Are the Options?

Before making a final decision to have a hysterectomy for endometriosis, you should know exactly what the procedure involves. A hysterectomy provides no guarantee of relief from the symptoms or from endometriosis. When a hysterectomy is performed and endometriosis is not entirely removed at the same time as the ovaries and uterus, there is a good chance that you may still have endometriosis after the hysterectomy.

In certain situations a hysterectomy may be warranted. However, before making any final decisions you should look into other less invasive alternatives for endometriosis. You should always get a second opinion before taking the final step. Reading personal stories and articles that have been written by women with endometriosis can be very helpful.

Join an endometriosis group, and discuss the various experiences other women have had after having a hysterectomy with endometriosis. Discuss possible side effects and risks with your doctor. And finally, carefully consider how you feel about having a hysterectomy for endometriosis, as this is not a reversible procedure.

Natural Treatments for Endometriosis

Endometriosis follows when the lining of the uterus attaches to surrounding tissues and organs causing variable degrees of pain and infertility. Selected herbal medicines can help provide relief as specific herbs help to re-balance the bodies hormone levels. There are also various herbal medicines that help strengthen the immune system and help combat disease. Endometriosis herbal medications, like all other alternative treatments involve a time commitment before success is achieved.

Herbal Remedies

• ProSmooth II a natural synergistic herbal formula has showed marked improvement for irritability, breast pain, pelvic cramps and pain, mood swings, headaches, uterine fibroids, weight gain and bloating. The formula comprises of vitex and dandelion that helps the body to eliminate excess external estrogen produced from hormone therapy and other environmental hormone disruptors such as xenosteriods.

• Bio identical progesterone helps to control endometriosis by reducing the estrogen effects on surrounding tissue. This option is now a recognized herbal treatment used to treat women with endometriosis.

• Evening Primrose provides a high content of GLA and phenylalanine which is being widely used to treat pain associated with endometriosis. GLA is essential for cell structure, improves nerve function and regulate hormone function. The oil helps reduce over stimulation of hormones, inflammation and lessens menstrual cramp.

Before selecting any natural remedies, therapy or changing your eating patterns, it is very important to consult with your medical practitioner.

Chapter 16: Overcome Endometriosis Without Gaining Weight

Women who suffer from endometriosis often find out that their condition is more problematic than they thought. Besides having to suffer from painful and heavy monthly periods, discomfort with sex and bowel movements, another possible negative side effect with endometriosis is weight gain. More and more women today are looking for ways to overcome endometriosis and it's troublesome side effects.

Endometriosis and Weight Gain

Few women realize that endometriosis treatment can lead to weight gain. This can be caused by three of the most popular types of medication used for treating endometriosis.

* Danazol -- The pituitary gland is one of the parts of the body that releases hormones. Danazol works by causing blockage to the production and release of FSH and LH hormones. This results to a temporary cease of your menstrual cycle that will last from a quarter to three-quarters of a year. Side effects include weight gain, oily skin and tiredness

* Birth Control Pills - Contraceptives can also work as a hormonal treatment to overcome endometriosis. The type and frequency of birth control pills that one should take will generally depend on your doctor's advice. Contraceptives work by regulating the progesterone and estrogen levels in your body. Again, this leads to a temporary stop to your monthly flow. If you choose to make this treatment permanent, your doctor might advise a gradual increase of frequency or dosage. Again weight gain is a side effect of this treatment, along with nausea and blood clots.

* Progestins - This medication results to a temporary stop to your ovulation and hinders growth of endometrial cells. This too comes with a number of side effects of which weight gain is one of them.

Prevent Weight Gain Caused by Medication

It's frustrating to women that the medicines that are supposed to help our symptoms also cause some unpleasant side effects. One of the most troublesome is the weight gain that often comes with the medication you're taking. Here are some things you can do to keep your weight under control.

Exercise

This may be a simple solution, and even an obvious one at that, but its effectiveness cannot be denied. Exercising can counter the weight gain side effect of your medication. Besides that, exercise can also reduce the severity of symptoms of endometriosis as it blocks the production of estrogen and releases endorphins into the system.

Change Medication

There are other hormonal treatments that you can take that don't have the weight gain side effect. Consider GnRH-agonists. These drugs treat endometriosis by releasing modified hormones that can stop production of estrogen and consequently cause a temporary cease to your menstrual cycle. The course of treatment lasts for around 6 months and the benefits can be felt for up to a further 6 months. Although weight gain is not a side effect there is the possibility of hot flashes, vaginal dryness and a loss of bone density during treatment, this is usually regained after stopping treatment.

Use of Natural Treatments

Of course, you also have the option of doing away with medical treatments all together and going for something more natural. You can treat endometriosis in a variety of ways such as taking herbal remedies, using stress-management and relaxation techniques, acupuncture, or contrast sitz baths. Talk to your doctor before stopping any prescribed treatment and inform them of your decision.

Modify Your Diet

If you wish to continue using the above-mentioned medication, you can still prevent yourself from gaining weight by proactively modifying your diet. Even if your medication does have this particular side effect, it won't be able to increase your weight too much if you're eating the right kinds of foods. Avoid eating processed, fried and sweet foods and chose a diet made up of fresh fruits and vegetables and lean meats and fish.

There are many ways for you to overcome endometriosis without gaining weight, but be aware that most of them will require some work on your part to keep your figure slim.

The Immune System and Endometriosis

Endometriosis is caused by series of cells forming within the uterus which are displaced. These cells remain in the uterus and grow and develop into painful adhesions. They are referred to by practitioners as retrograde cells.

After some research it was discovered that many woman actually experience these retrograde cells but were able to expel them quite easily thereby not developing the condition of Endometriosis. The main contributing factor why woman with Endometriosis are not able to expel these retrograde cells was a lowered immune system.

The immune system is lowered by many different factors within the body but the main contributor is found in the strength of the liver to overcome toxins and fight off diseases. When the liver is not functioning as it should be, the immune system is put under strain and is therefore not able to effectively fight off disease and toxins within the body.

It is the role of the liver to aid in breaking down proteins and nutrients from the foods that we eat. If the food we eat is not broken down effectively and incomplete digested food finds its way into the blood stream, it is then handled by the immune system. The toxins found within these foods can then damage the cells of the various body organs, including our uterus and cause inflammation.

Conclusion

It has been proven that many women with Endometriosis feel a significant improvement in their health and ability to cope with Endometriosis by simply increasing the immune fighting elements within the body. Immune fighting foods include high levels of anti-oxidants and foods which contain high levels of Vitamin C. Sugar is a large contributor in lowering the immune system and should be eliminated from the diet completely to allow the immune system to work at its best.

The immune system will benefit dramatically by building up the liver function through a liver cleansing technique or aiding the liver function. Dandelion Root and Milk Thistle are able to aid the liver function by increasing bile function, which is responsible for expelling waste products from the body.

Exercise is a strong focus when increasing the immune system as it is able to expel excess toxins through sweat and adequate movement in the body, creating blood flow. By increasing exercise to a daily 30 minute strategy, many women will experience dramatic improvement in both their immune system and ultimately the liver function.

We want to reduce any load on the liver through diet and exercise. We can reduce the work load on the liver by reducing medicated drugs, alcohol and caffeine. Choosing an easy to digest diet will naturally help the ability of the liver to cope with digestion.